METABOLIC CONFUSION DIET FOR SENIORS

Unlock Your Body's Potential for Health and Fitness Through Tasty Recipes, Meal Plans, and Simple Exercise for Long-Term Weight Loss and Healthy Aging

Vince Cruise Sant

Copyright © 2023

All Rights Are Reserved

The content in this book may not be reproduced, duplicated, or transferred without the express written permission of the author or publisher. Under no circumstances will the publisher or author be held liable or legally responsible for any losses, expenditures, or damages incurred directly or indirectly as a consequence of the information included in this book.

Legal Remarks

Copyright protection applies to this publication. It is only intended for personal use. No piece of this work may be modified, distributed, sold, quoted, or paraphrased without the author's or publisher's consent.

Disclaimer Statement

Please keep in mind that the contents of this booklet are meant for educational and recreational purposes. Every effort has been made to offer accurate, up-to-date, reliable, and thorough information. There are, however, no stated or implied assurances of any kind. Readers understand that the author is providing competent counsel. The content in this book originates from several sources. Please seek the opinion of a competent professional before using any of the tactics outlined in this book. By reading this book, the reader agrees that the author will not be held accountable for any direct or indirect damages resulting from the use of the information contained therein, including, but not limited to, errors, omissions, or inaccuracies.

TABLE OF CONTENTS

INTRODUCTION 6

Chapter One 10

Aging and Metabolism 10

    The Role of Metabolism in Aging 10

    Common Metabolic Changes in Seniors 13

    Importance of a Balanced Diet for Healthy Aging 16

Chapter Two 20

The Basics of Metabolic Confusion 20

    What is Metabolic Confusion? 20

    How Metabolic Confusion Differs from Other Diets .. 22

    Science Behind Metabolic Confusion for Seniors 25

Chapter Three 28

Getting Started 28

    Assessing Your Current Health and Diet 28

    Preparing Mentally and Emotionally 31

    Clearing Your Pantry and Shopping List Essentials . 34

Chapter Four 39

Phases of the Metabolic Confusion Diet 39

    Phase 1: Jumpstart Your Metabolism 39

Daily Meal Plans and Sample Recipes 42

Phase 2: Introducing Variation 47

Structuring Your Meals for Optimal Results 47

Adapting the Diet to Your Preferences..................50

Phase 3: Consolidation and Long-Term Success 52

Transitioning to a Sustainable Eating Pattern 52

Maintaining Results and Preventing Plateaus.......54

Chapter Five 58

Tailoring the Diet to Your Needs 58

Adapting Metabolic Confusion for Dietary Restrictions 58

Strategies for Overcoming Challenges....................61

Chapter Six 65

Lifestyle Factors for Enhanced Metabolism 65

Importance of Sleep for Metabolism.........................65

Managing Stress and Its Impact on Aging................68

Chapter Seven 73

Tracking Progress and Adjustments 73

Setting Realistic Goals for Health and Wellness 73

Identifying Plateaus and Making Necessary Changes 75

Chapter Eight 79

Long-Term Maintenance and Beyond 79

Transitioning to a Sustainable Dietary Pattern 79

Conclusion 82

INTRODUCTION

Welcome to "Metabolic Confusion Diet for Seniors," a thorough manual created to provide you with the information and resources you need to revitalize your metabolism, improve your wellbeing, and live out your golden years with fresh vigor. In these pages, we set out on a trip that combines cutting-edge research with doable tactics, designed especially for seniors looking to improve their health and lifespan.

Natural aging brings about a number of changes that have an effect on our bodies, including alterations in metabolism. The metabolic engine that once hummed regularly in our youth may progressively lose its effectiveness, posing problems such as trouble controlling weight, fluctuating energy levels, and an increased vulnerability to chronic illnesses. However, this is not where the narrative ends. The Metabolic Confusion Diet is a fantastic method for reigniting the metabolic fire inside.

The Metabolic Confusion Diet is a comprehensive method that uses the concepts of metabolic adaptability to rev up your body's energy production and illuminate your road to wellbeing. This book is your compass to navigate the diet. You may rouse your metabolism from its sleep, increase your energy levels, and produce sustained effects that go beyond the flimsy promises of fad diets by rotating between carefully tailored periods of eating and activity.

Starting a Transformational Journey

In the chapters that follow, we dig into the core of the Metabolic Confusion Diet, beginning with an examination of the relationship between aging and metabolism. The cornerstone of the specialized solutions that lie ahead is understanding the particular difficulties that elders encounter. We'll address misunderstandings about metabolic confusion and explain how it differs from other dietary approaches by exposing the science behind it.

We devote a portion to helping you psychologically and emotionally be ready, since the beginning of any transformational undertaking is sometimes the most difficult aspect. You'll be prepared to start your metabolic confusion quest with a clear head and unwavering resolve. Find out how to rid your pantry of potential hazards and adopt a shopping plan that promotes your health.

Following the Steps for Long-Term Success:

The three separate stages of the metabolic confusion diet are the focus of this book's core discussion. Phase 1 is where we kick-start your metabolism and lay the groundwork for a significant transformation. Sample menus and dishes will serve as a practical reference, and advice on how to exercise will help you achieve your objectives.

Phase 2 adds variety to keep your body on its toes and adjusting. Learn how to organize your meals for optimal impact and customize the diet to suit your interests and way of life. We'll support you in keeping up your workout schedule and walk you through more challenging metabolic exercises that may improve your outcomes even more.

Consolidation is important as we go towards Phase 3. This stage prepares you for a long-term lifestyle by avoiding plateaus and guaranteeing that your successes won't be fleeting. We'll go through how to keep up your renewed vigor and provide advice on how to make metabolic confusion principles a permanent part of your life.

A holistic strategy towards wellness

Beyond nutritional concerns, we explore lifestyle elements that work in concert to speed up your metabolism. An all-encompassing approach to well-being includes factors like getting enough sleep, controlling your stress, and being busy outside of regular exercise. Additionally, our meal planning and recipe area makes sure you have the useful resources to efficiently eat for your health.

A Pathway to Empowerment

The Metabolic Confusion Diet is a journey that involves more than simply physical change. It involves embracing your senior years with vigor and assurance. We urge you to keep track of your progress, establish reasonable objectives, and celebrate each success—not only on the scale but also in the way you feel, move, and live—throughout this book.

Remember that age is only a number as you begin this life-changing adventure and that your capacity for health has no limitations. Your friend, source of information, and vehicle for empowerment is "Metabolic Confusion Diet for Seniors". Together, let's open the doors to newfound vigor and write the next chapter of your active life.

CHAPTER ONE

AGING AND METABOLISM

The Role of Metabolism in Aging

Our bodies change as we age as a result of a complicated and varied process called metabolism, which plays a role in aging. The term metabolism refers to the totality of chemical activities and reactions that take place inside our cells to sustain life. Our bodies use it to transform food into energy, create and repair tissues, and control a number of physiological processes. Although metabolism is essential for maintaining life throughout our whole lifetime, as we get older, its dynamics alter, which may have an influence on a number of different elements of our health and wellbeing.

The following essential facts highlight the role metabolism plays in aging:

1. Energy use and calorie requirements: Our basal metabolic rate (BMR), which measures how much energy our body uses when at rest, tends to drop as we get older. Our bodies now need fewer calories to sustain essential processes like breathing, circulation, and cell repair. This is known as a decrease in BMR. If food choices are the same as they were in previous years, this lowered calorie need may lead to weight gain.

2. **Lean Muscle Mass:** Muscle mass tends to decline with age, a phenomenon known as sarcopenia. Muscle tissue is more metabolically active than fat tissue, meaning it burns more calories even when at rest. As muscle mass decreases, so does the body's capacity to burn calories, potentially leading to weight gain and changes in metabolism.

3. **Metabolic Rate Variability:** Although there is a general tendency toward a slower metabolic rate with aging, there is a lot of individual variation. The way one's metabolism evolves over time depends on a variety of variables, including genetics, lifestyle decisions, levels of physical activity, and general health.

4. **Hormonal Alterations:** Hormones are essential for controlling metabolism. Hormone sensitivity and production might change with aging. One possible effect is a drop in the levels of several hormones, including growth hormone, thyroid hormone, and sex hormones like estrogen and testosterone. The metabolism, body composition, and overall energy balance may all be impacted by these changes.

5. **Mitochondrial function and cellular aging:** The "powerhouses" of our cells, the mitochondria, are in charge of producing energy in the form of adenosine triphosphate (ATP). Oxidative stress and cumulative damage may cause mitochondrial function to deteriorate over time. Reduced energy generation and cellular efficiency may result from this, which may aggravate age-related health problems.

6. **Metabolic Stiffness:** Aging might result in a decreased capacity to adjust to variations in dietary consumption. This metabolic rigidity may make it more difficult to metabolize various foods and make you more vulnerable to insulin resistance, which is a major risk factor for type 2 diabetes.

7. **Inflammation and metabolism:** "Inflammation," or persistent low-grade inflammation, is linked to aging and may affect metabolism. Inflammatory activities may interfere with metabolic processes, which can impact insulin sensitivity and worsen metabolic syndrome and other age-related diseases.

For the purpose of encouraging healthy aging and addressing age-related health concerns, it is crucial to comprehend the function of metabolism in aging. Age-related metabolic changes may have detrimental impacts, although they can be somewhat mitigated by lifestyle choices including regular exercise, a nutritious diet, stress management, and enough sleep. People may work to preserve their metabolic health and general quality of life as they age by taking a holistic approach to well-being.

Common Metabolic Changes in Seniors

The variations that take place in the body's metabolic systems as individuals age are referred to as common metabolic changes in seniors. Numerous areas of health, including energy expenditure, nutritional consumption, hormone balance, and general wellbeing, might be impacted by these adjustments.

1. A decline in the basal metabolic rate (BMR): The amount of energy needed by the body to keep its essential processes running when at rest is known as the basal metabolic rate. Their BMR tends to decline as they get older. Because of this, the body burns fewer calories when at rest, which may result in weight gain if eating habits are not modified appropriately.

2. Decrease in lean muscle mass: The age-related decrease of muscle mass and strength, known as sarcopenia, plays a crucial role in the metabolic alterations that occur in older people. Since muscle tissue has a higher metabolic rate than fat tissue, it burns more calories. The body's capacity to burn calories declines when muscle mass declines, potentially resulting in weight gain and decreased metabolic effectiveness.

3. **Reduction in Physical Activity:** Many seniors experience a decline in physical activity as a result of mobility issues, chronic illnesses, or lifestyle modifications. Less physical activity may exacerbate muscle loss, a decline in BMR, and changes to metabolism.

4. **Hormonal Alterations:** Hormones are essential for controlling metabolism. Age-related alterations in hormone sensitivity and production are possible. For instance, the decline in sex hormones (estrogen and testosterone) may have an impact on muscular mass, bone density, and fat distribution. Additionally, a drop in thyroid hormone levels might impact metabolic rate.

5. **Insulin Sensitivity and Glucose Regulation**: As we get older, it's more common to develop insulin resistance, which affects the body's capacity to react to insulin and control blood sugar levels. Greater blood sugar levels, a

greater risk of type 2 diabetes, and metabolic syndrome may result from this.

6. **Modifications to the Fat Distribution:** In particular, visceral fat, or the fat surrounding organs, may grow and subcutaneous fat, or the fat beneath the skin, may decrease as people age. An increased risk of metabolic diseases and cardiovascular disease is linked to this change.

7. **Digestive System Changes:** The digestive system can undergo changes with age, affecting nutrient absorption and metabolism. Reduced stomach acid production and changes in gut microbiota composition can impact nutrient absorption, potentially leading to deficiencies.

8. **Mitochondrial Activity:** Mitochondria, the organelles in cells that provide energy, may become less effective and functional as they get older. Reduced energy generation and a general metabolic slowdown may result from this.

9. **Inflammation and Oxidative Stress:** Chronic low-grade inflammation and oxidative stress increase with age, affecting metabolic pathways and potentially

contributing to insulin resistance, metabolic syndrome, and other age-related conditions.

10. **Kidney function and hydration:** Due to changes in thirst perception and renal function, dehydration becomes more prevalent in older people. For metabolic processes to remain stable, proper hydration is necessary.

11. **Drug Interactions:** Seniors often take many medicines, and certain drugs might affect nutritional interactions and metabolism. When prescribing drugs for elderly patients, healthcare professionals should take these variables into account.

Understanding these typical metabolic alterations in older people emphasizes the need for a thorough strategy for healthy aging. The best metabolic health may be supported in older persons by engaging in regular physical exercise, eating a nutritious diet, preserving muscle mass via strength training, treating chronic illnesses, and drinking enough water.

Importance of a Balanced Diet for Healthy Aging

In order to maintain general wellbeing and lessen the consequences of age-related changes, a balanced diet is essential for supporting healthy aging. It provides the essential nutrients, energy, and components. An individual's dietary requirements may change as they age, making a well-balanced diet even more important for preserving good health. A balanced diet is crucial for good aging for the following main reasons:

1. Intake of Nutrients: Seniors who follow a balanced diet are certain to get the vital elements they need, including vitamins, minerals, proteins, carbs, lipids, and fiber. These vitamins and minerals are essential for preserving biological processes, bolstering the immune system, encouraging cellular repair, and avoiding shortages that may cause a number of health problems.

2. Muscular Size and Strength: It's essential to consume enough protein to maintain muscle mass and strength, which is particularly crucial to avoiding sarcopenia (age-related muscle loss). Protein helps muscles develop, mend, and function as a whole, keeping elders mobile and independent.

3. Bone Health: A balanced diet rich in calcium and vitamin D is critical for maintaining bone health and reducing the risk of osteoporosis. Adequate calcium and vitamin D intake help support bone density and prevent fractures, which can be more common in older adults.

4. Cardiovascular health: A heart-healthy diet that is balanced and abundant in whole grains, fiber, and heart-healthy fats (such as omega-3 fatty acids) may help maintain cardiovascular health. This may assist in lowering the risk of heart disease, hypertension, and stroke.

5. Cognitive Function: Some nutrients, including antioxidants (vitamins C and E), omega-3 fatty acids, and B vitamins, have been associated with good cognitive health. These nutrients may promote healthy brain function and contribute to a balanced diet that can help prevent cognitive decline.

6. Control of Blood Sugar: A healthy diet rich in lean proteins, fiber, and complex carbs may help control blood sugar levels and lower the risk of type 2 diabetes. Seniors must manage their blood sugar in particular since they may be more prone to insulin resistance.

7. Digestive Health: A diet high in fiber from fruits, vegetables, whole grains, and legumes improves digestive health by encouraging regular bowel movements and reducing constipation, a problem that is frequent in older people.

8. Immune System Support: Proper nutrition supports the immune system's ability to fight infections and illnesses. Nutrients such as vitamins A, C, and E, as well as zinc and selenium, play essential roles in immune function.

9. Managing Your Weight: Seniors may maintain a healthy weight with the aid of a balanced diet. It supplies the required energy for everyday tasks while assisting in preventing excessive weight gain, which may cause a number of health issues.

10. Energy and Vitality: Consuming a range of nutrient-dense meals gives you the energy you need for everyday tasks and helps you stay awake by preventing weariness, improving your general vitality and quality of life.

11. Reduced Risk of Chronic Diseases: A balanced diet can help reduce the risk of chronic diseases such as heart disease, diabetes, and certain types of cancer, which become more prevalent with age.

12. Mental and emotional health: Omega-3 fatty acids and certain vitamins are among the nutritional components that have been linked to improved mood and mental health. A balanced diet may support both emotional and cognitive health.

CHAPTER TWO

THE BASICS OF METABOLIC CONFUSION

What is Metabolic Confusion?

A diet and exercise technique called metabolic confusion, often referred to as the metabolic confusion diet or metabolic cycling, is used to increase the body's metabolism by varying the number of calories consumed, the proportion of macronutrients consumed, and the amount of activity performed. The purpose of metabolic confusion is to stop the body from becoming used to a certain food and exercise regimen, which might result in weight loss or fitness improvement plateaus.

The premise that the body tends to adapt to regular patterns over time is the foundation of the concept of metabolic confusion. If you stick to the same eating plan and exercise routine for a long time, your metabolism may become more adept at using calories and nutrients, which may slow down weight loss or muscle growth. By introducing fluctuations in calorie intake, nutritional ratios, and exercise intensity, metabolic confusion seeks to impair this adaptation process.

The normal process of metabolic confusion is as follows:

1. **Caloric variability:** Metabolic confusion entails switching between days of greater and lower caloric consumption as opposed to constantly eating the same number of calories each day. It is believed that this variety prevents the body from becoming used to a regular energy supply.

2. **Cycles of macronutrients:** Carbohydrates, proteins, and fats may be distributed differently on various days or periods of the diet. For instance, some days could concentrate on eating more carbs, while others would emphasize eating more protein or healthy fats.

3. **Alternate-Day Fasting:** Metabolic confusion may include intermittent fasting, which alternates between eating and not eating. This may stimulate the body to utilize stored energy and help control insulin levels.

4. **Exercise Alternative:** Exercise for metabolic confusion entails varying the kind, level, and length of exercises. By preventing muscles from responding, this may encourage ongoing muscular development and fat burning.

5. Mealtimes and Routine: Eating habits may also change, with some days emphasizing a few, bigger meals while others focus on many, smaller meals. This strategy may avoid metabolic adaptation by keeping the body guessing.

6. The cycle phases People who have metabolic confusion often choose a cyclical strategy, cycling through various calorie intake, macronutrient distribution, and activity stages over predetermined time periods, such as weekly or monthly cycles.

Although metabolic confusion may seem promising, there is not much evidence to support its efficacy in the scientific community. The strategy is based on the ideas of metabolic adaptability and variation in food and exercise, but further study is required to establish its long-term effectiveness, safety, and suitability for use with various populations.

How Metabolic Confusion Differs from Other Diets

In comparison to previous diets, metabolic confusion takes a different approach to weight reduction and metabolic adaptation. While many diets concentrate on certain calorie limits, macronutrient ratios, or dietary limitations, metabolic confusion seeks to stop the body from becoming used to one particular eating and activity pattern. The following is how metabolic confusion differs from other diet strategies:

1. Variability and Cycling: Metabolic confusion revolves around the idea of introducing variation into diet and exercise patterns. Instead of following a static set of rules, metabolic confusion involves cycling through different phases of caloric intake, macronutrient distribution, exercise intensity, and even meal timing. This variation is thought to prevent the body from plateauing and adapting to a fixed routine.

2. Avoiding Adaptation: The goal of metabolic confusion is to keep the body "confused" by often switching its inputs, in contrast to certain conventional diets that might cause metabolic adaptation (where the body gets more effective at using fewer calories). Theoretically, this helps avoid the metabolic slowing that might result from prolonged calorie restriction.

3. The Cyclical Nature: Individuals who have metabolic disorientation often cycle through many stages. This may take the form of weekly or monthly cycles, with each phase concentrating on certain dietary and exercise-related topics. For instance, one phase can concentrate on consuming more calories and carbohydrates, while another would focus on consuming fewer calories and engaging in more strenuous activity.

4. **Exercise Accentuation:** Traditional diets may put a strong emphasis on calorie intake and the ratios of different macronutrients, while metabolic confusion places a strong emphasis on exercise variety. The body is less likely to adapt to a particular exercise regimen when the kind, intensity, and length of exercises are varied.

5. **Customization:** Metabolic confusion allows for greater customization based on individual preferences and responses. People can tailor their phases of higher and lower caloric intake, macronutrient distribution, and exercise intensity to suit their goals and lifestyle.

6. **Long-Term Adjustment:** The goal of metabolic confusion is to provide a long-term method of weight control, in contrast to those diets that are intended for quick effects. Proponents of metabolic confusion contend that it may be a long-term weight reduction method since it avoids adaptation and plateaus.

Although the idea of metabolic confusion has drawn interest, there has only been a limited amount of scientific study testing its efficacy and safety in comparison to other dietary regimens. Individual outcomes may differ with any diet plan, and there may be dangers or difficulties brought on by frequent changes in calorie intake and food distribution.

Science Behind Metabolic Confusion for Seniors

The "science" behind metabolic confusion in seniors is based on a number of interrelated physiological principles and ideas, however it's crucial to highlight that this methodology hasn't been thoroughly investigated or supported by solid scientific study. The core concepts are based on how the body adjusts to dietary, physical activity, and metabolic changes. The following are some crucial ideas that supporters of metabolic confusion often stress:

1. Metabolic Adjustment: The body is remarkably capable of adjusting to dietary and exercise changes. This may result in metabolic adaptation, when the body improves its capacity to use food and energy. This may cause a weight reduction or fitness improvement plateau over time.

2. Variability Disruption: By often changing calorie intake, the distribution of macronutrients, and exercise intensity, metabolic confusion tries to interfere with this adaptation. According to the notion, if the body is repeatedly exposed to novel stimuli, it will have a harder time adapting.

3. Hormonal Reaction: Hormonal responses may be changed by altering calorie intake and the distribution of macronutrients. Changing between periods of greater and reduced carbohydrate consumption, for instance, might affect insulin levels and other hormones that affect metabolism and hunger.

4. Exercise Results: The body can't become proficient at certain actions and muscle groups if the kind, intensity, and length of training regimens are changed often. This may encourage the development of lean muscle, the burning of fat, and general fitness gains.

5. Insulin Sensitivity: Insulin sensitivity is hypothesized to be affected by several variables within metabolic confusion, such as intermittent fasting or cycling carbohydrate consumption. Enhancing insulin sensitivity may help with weight reduction goals and improve blood sugar management.

6. **Adaptation of the mitochondria:** Mitochondrial adaptations may be impacted by metabolic disarray. Supporters of this strategy claim that it may promote mitochondrial efficiency and function by routinely altering energy demands via adjustments in exercise intensity and nutrition intake.

7. **Preventing Plateaus:** The cyclical nature of metabolic confusion is designed to prevent plateaus by keeping the body "guessing." This constant variation aims to maintain a level of metabolic challenge that supports ongoing progress.

Despite the fact that these ideas seem reasonable, it's critical to point out that there is a dearth of research on metabolic confusion, particularly in relation to elderly people. Few research has looked explicitly at the effects of metabolic confusion diets, especially in older persons. Instead of being supported by solid scientific data, the majority of the assertions are based on hypothetical reasoning and anecdotal accounts.

CHAPTER THREE

GETTING STARTED

Assessing Your Current Health and Diet

Before making any dietary or lifestyle changes, including strategies like the metabolic confusion diet, it is essential to evaluate your current health and diet. A comprehensive evaluation offers insightful information about your starting position, indicates possible improvement areas, and helps in the development of a customized plan that is in line with your objectives and medical requirements. Here's how to accurately evaluate your present diet and health:

1. Medical Background and Current Health Status:

- Get a thorough physical examination to determine your starting point for wellness.

2. Nutritional Analysis:

- For a few days, record your meals and liquid intake in a food diary. Include meal times and portion quantities.
- To examine your nutritional consumption, including calories, macronutrients (carbohydrates,

proteins, and fats), vitamins, and minerals, use online tools or applications.

3. **Body Composition:**
   - Determine your weight and, if feasible, the proportion of body fat. This might help you gain an understanding of your body's composition and possible areas for growth.

4. **Blood Work:**
   - Think about obtaining blood testing to check your blood pressure, fasting glucose, and other pertinent indicators.
   - If necessary, discuss testing that might shed light on vitamin inadequacies with your healthcare professional.

5. **Physical Activity:**
   - Assess your degree of physical activity right now. Keep track of the kind, frequency, and force of your exercises or other activities.
   - Evaluate your cardiovascular fitness, strength, and flexibility.

6. Sleep and Stress:

- Consider your slumber habits and general quality of sleep. Sleep deprivation may affect metabolism and general health.
- Think about your stress levels and coping mechanisms. Chronic stress may have an impact on well-being and weight control.

7. Dietary Preferences and Allergies:

- List any dietary intolerances or allergies you may have.
- Recognize your nutritional needs and preferences, as well as any cultural or ethnic constraints.

8. Health Goals

- Clearly state your health objectives. Are you trying to lose weight, increase muscle, have more energy, have better blood sugar management, or just be healthier overall?

9. Lifestyle Factors:

- Take into account elements like your daily schedule, employment, and social obligations that might affect your food preferences and meal times.

10. Mindset and Motivation:

- Consider whether you're open to change. What inspires you to enhance your diet and physical fitness? Are you prepared to make changes?

You'll obtain a detailed grasp of your starting position and the areas where you may make changes by carefully evaluating your current diet and health. Regardless of whether you choose for a metabolic confusion method or another dietary strategy, this knowledge will assist you in creating a personalized plan that takes into consideration your unique requirements, preferences, and health objectives.

Preparing Mentally and Emotionally

Making sustained adjustments to your food and lifestyle, especially strategies like the metabolic confusion diet, requires careful mental and emotional preparation. It entails developing the appropriate mentality, establishing reasonable expectations, and fostering the psychological resilience required to overcome obstacles and remain dedicated to your objectives.

1. Set clear goals: Clearly state your objectives for your health and wellbeing. Having clear objectives will help you stay motivated and focused, whether your objective is weight reduction, increased fitness, more energy, or general well-being.

2. Understand Your "Why": Determine the causes of your desire to modify your diet. Knowing what drives you will provide you with a solid foundation and serve as a constant reminder of the advantages you're pursuing.

3. Adopt a positive outlook: Develop an optimistic, growth-oriented mentality. Accept the notion that change takes time and that obstacles are a normal part of the path. Place more emphasis on growth than on perfection.

4. Visualize Success: Imagine attaining your objectives. Imagine how your life will change, how you will feel, and how your health will improve. This mental image helps solidify your resolve and motivate you to take action.

5. Manage Expectations: Be aware that outcomes may not manifest right away. Setting reasonable goals and being patient with your efforts can help you make lasting improvements.

6. Establish a Helpful Environment: Embrace those who will help you achieve your objectives. Tell your loved ones about your goals so they can support you and hold you accountable.

7. Develop Coping Strategies: Determine any obstacles or triggers that could stand in the way of your advancement. Create coping mechanisms for stressful situations, emotional eating, and temptations.

8. Educate yourself on self-compassion: Be kind to yourself and work on this. Recognize that setbacks sometimes occur, but instead of using them as an excuse to quit, utilize them as learning opportunities.

9. Honor little victories: Celebrate all achievements, no matter how little. Celebrate your victories along the way to keep yourself inspired and upbeat.

10. Mindful Consumption: By observing your hunger signals, enjoying each meal, and eating without interruptions, you may practice mindful eating. Healthy dietary habits promote a better relationship with food.

11. Stay informed: Continue your education in the areas of food, exercise, and the fundamentals of the metabolic confusion diet. Your dedication may be strengthened if you know the "why" behind your decisions.

12. Practice stress management: Take part in activities you find relaxing, such as deep breathing exercises, yoga, meditation, or hobbies. It's crucial to manage stress if you want to maintain your emotional health.

13. Maintain flexibility: Be willing to modify your strategy in light of your experiences. Don't be afraid to make changes if something isn't operating as it should.

14. Follow Your Progress: Use an app or a diary to record your progress. You can observe how far you've come and see trends that contribute to your success by keeping a journal of your trip.

15. Professional Guidance: If necessary, look for assistance from specialists in behavior modification and mental well-being, such as therapists, counselors, or registered dietitians.

The ongoing process of mentally and emotionally preparing calls for self-awareness, self-compassion, and a dedication to your well-being. You'll be better able to overcome obstacles, maintain consistency, and bring about the desired changes if you lay a solid foundation of emotional and mental fortitude.

Clearing Your Pantry and Shopping List Essentials

Clearing your pantry and creating a shopping list of essentials are important steps in adopting a new dietary approach like the metabolic confusion diet. These steps help you create an environment that supports your health goals and ensures that you have the right foods on hand to follow your chosen plan effectively. Here's how to clear your pantry and prepare a shopping list:

Clearing Your Pantry:

1. **Remove temptations:** Identify foods that don't align with your new dietary goals. This may include processed snacks, sugary foods, unhealthy oils, and high-calorie treats. Remove these items from your pantry to reduce temptation.

2. **Check Expiry Dates:** Go through your pantry and discard any expired or stale foods. Keeping fresh ingredients is essential for preparing nutritious meals.

3. **Donate or Give Away:** If you have non-perishable items that you won't be consuming, consider donating them to a food bank or giving them to friends and family who might find them useful.

4. **Organize:** After removing unwanted items, organize your pantry to make healthy choices more accessible. Place nutritious foods at eye level and keep less healthy options hidden or out of reach.

Creating a Shopping List of Essentials

1. **Fresh Produce:** Include a variety of fruits and vegetables. Choose different colors to ensure a diverse range of vitamins, minerals, and antioxidants.

Leafy greens, berries, citrus fruits, cruciferous vegetables, and root vegetables are excellent options.

2. **Lean Proteins:** opt for lean protein sources such as skinless poultry, lean cuts of meat, fish, tofu, tempeh, legumes (beans, lentils, chickpeas), and low-fat dairy or dairy alternatives.

3. **Whole Grains:** Choose whole grains like brown rice, quinoa, oats, whole wheat pasta, and whole grain bread. These provide complex carbohydrates and fiber.

4. **Healthy Fats:** Include sources of healthy fats like avocados, nuts, seeds, olive oil, and fatty fish (salmon, mackerel, and sardines) rich in omega-3 fatty acids.

5. **Dairy and Dairy Alternatives:** Select low-fat or Greek yogurt, skim milk, or dairy alternatives like almond milk or soy milk.

6. **Nuts and Seeds:** Stock up on a variety of nuts (almonds, walnuts, pistachios) and seeds (chia seeds,

flaxseeds, sunflower seeds) to add texture and nutrition to meals.

7. **Herbs and Spices:** Enhance flavor without adding excess calories by using a variety of herbs and spices such as basil, oregano, cinnamon, turmeric, and ginger.

8. **Condiments and Sauces:** Choose low-sodium soy sauce, vinegar, salsa, mustard, and other flavor-enhancing condiments.

9. **Healthy Snacks:** Include options like fresh fruit, vegetable sticks with hummus, Greek yogurt, or a handful of nuts for satisfying between-meal snacks.

10. **Hydration:** Stock up on water and herbal teas to stay hydrated throughout the day.

11. **Meal Plan Ingredients**: Consider the recipes you'll be preparing and add any specific ingredients required for your metabolic confusion meal plan.

12. **Shopping Tips:** Prioritize whole, unprocessed foods.

- Choose fresh produce in season for optimal flavor and nutrient content.
- Read food labels to make informed choices about packaged foods.

- Shop the perimeter of the grocery store for fresh foods and minimize processed items in the center aisles.

By clearing your pantry of foods that don't align with your goals and creating a shopping list filled with nutritious essentials, you're setting yourself up for success in adopting the metabolic confusion diet or any other dietary approach you choose. Remember to plan ahead, shop mindfully, and enjoy the process of nourishing your body with wholesome foods.

CHAPTER FOUR

PHASES OF THE METABOLIC CONFUSION DIET

Phase 1: Jumpstart Your Metabolism

Phase 1 of the metabolic confusion diet is designed to jumpstart your metabolism by introducing specific dietary and exercise changes. This phase typically involves higher caloric intake, specific macronutrient ratios, and targeted exercises to create a metabolic shift. The goal is to prevent adaptation, encourage metabolic responsiveness, and set the stage for sustainable progress. Keep in mind that the specific details of Phase 1 can vary based on individual preferences and needs. Here's a general outline of Phase 1:

Dietary Changes:

1. Caloric Increase: During Phase 1, you'll increase your caloric intake compared to your baseline. This caloric increase aims to counteract potential metabolic adaptations from prior calorie restriction.

2. Carbohydrate Emphasis: Carbohydrates are prioritized in this phase to provide energy and support metabolic responsiveness. Include whole grains, fruits, vegetables, and legumes in your meals.

3. **Protein Intake:** Maintain a moderate protein intake to support muscle preservation and recovery from exercise. Lean protein sources like poultry, fish, lean meats, tofu, and legumes are good choices.

4. **Healthy Fats:** Include healthy fats like avocados, nuts, seeds, and olive oil to support satiety and overall well-being.

5. **Meal Frequency:** Spread your caloric intake across multiple meals and snacks throughout the day. This helps regulate blood sugar levels and prevents extreme hunger.

6. **Hydration:** Stay well-hydrated by drinking water throughout the day. Herbal teas and other non-caloric beverages can also be included.

Exercise Changes:

1. **Strength Training:** Focus on strength training exercises that target major muscle groups. This can stimulate muscle growth and boost metabolism.

2. **Higher reps, lower weight:** During Phase 1, you might opt for higher repetitions with slightly lower weights. This

approach can contribute to muscle endurance and engagement.

3. **Cardiovascular Exercise:** Incorporate cardiovascular activities like brisk walking, cycling, or swimming to enhance overall fitness and calorie expenditure.

4. **Variation:** Change up your exercise routine regularly to prevent the body from adapting. This might involve rotating between different exercises, intensities, and modalities.

Supplements and Support:

1. **Nutrient help:** Consider supplements that may help your metabolic objectives, such as omega-3 fatty acids, vitamins, and minerals. However, focus on obtaining nutrients primarily from whole foods.

Monitoring Progress:

1. **Measurements:** Track changes in weight, body measurements, and how your clothes fit to monitor progress.

2. **Energy Levels:** Notice changes in your energy levels, mood, and general well-being. Positive swings in energy might signal that your metabolism is reacting effectively.

Daily Meal Plans and Sample Recipes

Day 1: Higher Caloric Intake, Carbohydrate Emphasis

Breakfast:
- Scrambled Eggs with Spinach and Tomatoes
- Whole-Grain Toast
- Sliced avocado

Lunch:
- Grilled Chicken Salad with Mixed Greens, Bell Peppers, Cucumbers, and Quinoa
- Olive Oil and Balsamic Vinegar Dressing

Afternoon Snack:
- Greek Yogurt with Berries and a Drizzle of Honey

Dinner:
- Baked Salmon with Lemon and Herbs
- Steamed Broccoli
- Brown Rice

Day 2: Strength Training and Cardiovascular Exercise

Breakfast:
- Oatmeal with Almond Butter, Chopped Nuts, and Banana Slices

Lunch:

- Turkey and Hummus Wrap with Whole Wheat Tortilla, Mixed Greens, and Sliced Veggies

Afternoon Snack:

Carrot Sticks with Hummus

Dinner:

- Stir-Fried Tofu and Mixed Vegetables in Teriyaki Sauce
- Quinoa

Day 3: Higher Protein Intake

Breakfast:

- Greek Yogurt Parfait with Granola and Mixed Berries

Lunch:

- lentil and vegetable soup
- Whole Grain Roll

Afternoon Snack:

- Cottage Cheese with Pineapple Chunks

Dinner: Grilled Steak with Roasted Sweet Potatoes and Asparagus

As you create your meal plans, consider the principles of Phase 1, such as higher caloric intake, carbohydrate emphasis, and strength training exercises. You can modify portion sizes, ingredient choices, and meal times to suit your schedule and preferences. Additionally, consulting with a registered dietitian or nutrition professional can provide personalized guidance and help you create meal plans that align with your goals and needs.

Recipes

Sample Recipe 1: Scrambled Eggs with Spinach and Tomatoes

Ingredients:

- 2 eggs
- Handful of baby spinach
- 1 small tomato, diced
- Salt and pepper to taste
- Olive oil or cooking spray

Instructions:

1. Heat a non-stick skillet over medium heat and add a small amount of olive oil or cooking spray.

2. In a bowl, whisk the eggs and season with salt and pepper.

3. Pour the whisked eggs into the skillet and let them cook for a minute until they start to set.

4. Add the diced tomatoes and baby spinach to the eggs.

5. Gently scramble the mixture with a spatula until the eggs are fully cooked and the spinach is wilted.

6. Transfer the scrambled eggs to a plate and serve with whole-grain toast and sliced avocado.

Sample Recipe 2: Grilled Chicken Salad with Quinoa
Ingredients:

- 4 oz. grilled chicken breast, sliced
- Mixed greens (lettuce, spinach, arugula)
- 1/4 cup cooked quinoa
- Sliced bell peppers
- Sliced cucumbers
- Olive oil and balsamic vinegar for dressing

Instructions: 1. Arrange the mixed greens on a plate.

2. Top with grilled chicken slices, cooked quinoa, bell peppers, and cucumbers.

3. Drizzle olive oil and balsamic vinegar as a dressing.

4. Toss the salad gently to combine the ingredients.

5. Enjoy the flavorful and filling salad as a balanced and nutritious meal.

Sample Recipe 3: Oatmeal with Almond Butter and Banana

Ingredients:

- 1/2 cup rolled oats
- 1 cup water or milk of choice
- 1 tablespoon almond butter
- 1 banana, sliced
- Chopped nuts (optional)

Instructions:

1. In a saucepan, bring the water or milk to a boil.

2. Stir in the rolled oats and reduce the heat to a simmer.

3. Cook the oats, stirring occasionally, until they reach your desired consistency (usually about 5-7 minutes).

4. Transfer the cooked oatmeal to a bowl.

5. Top the oatmeal with almond butter, sliced banana, and chopped nuts if desired.

6. Mix everything together and enjoy a warm and satisfying breakfast.

Phase 2: Introducing Variation

Structuring Your Meals for Optimal Results

Structuring your meals for optimal results in the context of the metabolic confusion diet involves carefully planning your nutrition to support your goals, maintain energy levels, and prevent metabolic adaptation. Here's how you can effectively structure your meals for success:

1. Balance Macronutrients:

- Each meal should include a balance of carbohydrates, proteins, and healthy fats.
- Carbohydrates provide energy, proteins support muscle repair and growth, and healthy fats contribute to satiety and overall well-being.

2. Portion Control:

- Pay attention to portion sizes to avoid overeating.
- Use visual cues like your hand to estimate portion sizes of protein, carbohydrates, and fats.

3. Timing of Meals:

- Space your meals and snacks throughout the day to maintain steady energy levels and prevent extreme hunger.

- Aim for three main meals and one to two snacks, as needed.

4. Post-Workout Nutrition:

- Consume a combination of carbohydrates and proteins after workouts to support muscle recovery and replenish glycogen stores.

5. High-Quality Carbohydrates:

- Focus on complex carbohydrates like whole grains, fruits, and vegetables.
- These provide sustained energy and essential nutrients.

6. Lean Proteins:

- Choose lean protein sources like poultry, fish, lean meats, tofu, legumes, and low-fat dairy.
- Protein supports muscle maintenance and growth, along with a feeling of fullness.

7. Healthy Fats:

- Incorporate healthy fats from sources like avocados, nuts, seeds, and olive oil.
- Fats support hormone production and help you feel satisfied.

8. Fiber-Rich Foods:

- Include fiber-rich foods like vegetables, fruits, whole grains, and legumes.
- Fiber promotes digestion, helps control appetite, and supports gut health.

9. Hydration:

- Drink water throughout the day to stay hydrated.
- Hydration is essential for overall health and metabolism.

10. Limit Added Sugars:

- Minimize foods and beverages high in added sugars.
- opt for naturally sweet options like whole fruits.

11. Variety:

- Aim for a variety of foods to ensure you get a wide range of nutrients.
- Experiment with different foods to keep meals interesting.

12. Plan Ahead:

- Plan your meals and snacks in advance to make healthy choices easier.

- Prepare meals and snacks in batches for convenience.

13. Mindful Eating:
- Practice mindful eating by eating slowly, savoring flavors, and paying attention to hunger and fullness cues.

14. Listen to Your Body:
- Adjust your meal structure based on how your body responds. Everyone's needs are unique.

Remember that individual needs and preferences vary, so it's important to personalize your meal structure to align with your lifestyle and objectives. The key is to nourish your body with balanced, nutrient-dense meals that support your metabolic health and overall well-being.

Adapting the Diet to Your Preferences

Adapting the metabolic confusion diet to your preferences is essential for long-term success and sustainability. While the core principles of the diet focus on introducing variation, maintaining a balanced diet, and preventing metabolic adaptation, there's room for flexibility to suit your individual tastes, dietary restrictions, and lifestyle. Here's how you can adapt the diet to your preferences:

1. Choose foods you enjoy: Incorporate foods you love that align with the principles of the diet. This makes it easier to stick to the plan.

2. Customize Macronutrient Ratios: Within the framework of the diet, adjust the proportions of carbohydrates, proteins, and fats to match your preferences and dietary needs.

3. Explore Culinary Creativity: Experiment with different cooking methods, flavors, and cuisines to keep your meals interesting and enjoyable.

4. Substitute Ingredients: If you have food allergies, sensitivities, or dietary restrictions, find suitable substitutions for specific ingredients in the recipes.

5. Meal Timing: Adjust meal timing to fit your schedule and preferences. Focus on consistency in timing to regulate your metabolism.

6. Dietary Restrictions: If you follow specific dietary patterns (e.g., vegetarian, vegan, or gluten-free), adapt recipes to accommodate your preferences.

7. Portion Sizes: Tailor portion sizes to your hunger and activity level. Avoid overly strict calorie counting if it doesn't align with your preferences.

8. Intuitive Eating: Listen to your body's hunger and fullness cues to guide your eating patterns.

9. Experiment with Phases: Test different variations in the phases of the diet to find what works best for you.

10. Indulge Mindfully: Allow yourself occasional treats or favorite foods in moderation, practicing mindfulness while enjoying them.

11. Stay Adaptable: Be open to adjusting the diet based on your evolving preferences, goals, and feedback from your body.

12. Gradual Changes: If the diet feels overwhelming, start with gradual changes to ease into the new eating pattern.

Remember that the primary goal is to create a balanced and sustainable approach that supports your health and well-being. By tailoring the metabolic confusion diet to your preferences, you're more likely to enjoy the journey and achieve lasting results that fit your unique lifestyle.

Phase 3: Consolidation and Long-Term Success

Transitioning to a Sustainable Eating Pattern

Transitioning to a sustainable eating pattern after following the metabolic confusion diet involves finding a balance between your health goals, dietary preferences, and long-term well-being.

1. **Reflect on Your Experience:** Take time to reflect on your experience with the metabolic confusion diet. What aspects worked well for you? What did you enjoy, and what challenges did you face?

2. **Identify sustainable habits:** Identify the dietary and lifestyle habits that you found sustainable and enjoyable. These are the practices you can incorporate into your long-term eating pattern.

3. **Focus on Whole Foods:** Emphasize whole foods in your diet. Incorporate a variety of fruits, vegetables, lean proteins, whole grains, and healthy fats.

4. **Listen to Your Body:** Pay attention to your body's hunger and fullness cues. Eat when you're hungry, and stop when you're satisfied.

5. **Choose balanced meals:** Continue to create balanced meals that include a combination of carbohydrates, proteins, and fats. This promotes steady energy levels and overall health.

6. **Include foods you love:** Integrate your favorite foods into your eating pattern. Enjoying meals, you love helps make your diet sustainable.

7. Portion Control: Practice portion control to prevent overeating. Use mindful eating techniques to savor your meals.

8. Plan Ahead: Plan your meals and snacks ahead of time to make healthy choices convenient.

9. Be Flexible: Allow yourself flexibility to enjoy special occasions and occasional treats without guilt.

10. Incorporate Variety: Include a variety of foods to ensure you're getting a wide range of nutrients. Experiment with different recipes and cuisines.

11. Gradual Adjustments: Transition slowly and gradually. Make small adjustments over time rather than completely overhauling your eating pattern.

12. Monitor Progress: Regularly assess how you feel, your energy levels, and any changes in your body composition.

13. Be patient and kind to yourself: Embrace the process of finding a sustainable eating pattern that fits your lifestyle and promotes your health.

Maintaining Results and Preventing Plateaus

Maintaining results and preventing plateaus after following the metabolic confusion diet requires ongoing commitment, smart strategies, and a focus on sustainable habits. Here's how to maintain your progress and continue making positive changes:

1. Embrace a Healthy Lifestyle: Shift your mindset from a short-term diet to a lifelong commitment to health. Focus on making sustainable lifestyle changes.

2. Continuously Vary Your Routine: Continue to incorporate variation into your exercise routine. Change up your workouts, intensity, and types of activities regularly.

3. Adjust Caloric Intake: As your body changes, adjust your caloric intake to match your energy needs. Consult a professional for guidance if needed.

4. Gradual Changes: Make gradual adjustments to your eating pattern and exercise routine to avoid sudden shifts that can lead to plateaus.

5. Mindful Eating: Practice mindful eating to become attuned to your body's hunger and fullness cues. Avoid overeating or undereating.

6. Strength Training: Continue incorporating strength training to maintain muscle mass, boost metabolism, and support bone health.

7. Set New Goals: Establish new fitness and health goals to keep yourself motivated and engaged in your journey.

8. Monitor Progress: Regularly assess your progress through measurements, body composition analysis, and performance improvements.

9. Stay Hydrated: Keep drinking plenty of water to support metabolism, digestion, and overall health.

10. Prioritize Sleep: Aim for adequate sleep to support recovery, energy levels, and hormonal balance.

11. Celebrate non-scale victories: Focus on non-scale victories such as increased strength, improved endurance, and enhanced overall well-being.

12. Intuitive Eating: Listen to your body's cues and eat in response to physical hunger rather than emotional triggers.

13. Consistency is Key: Stick to your chosen eating pattern and exercise routine consistently over time to maintain results.

14. Regular Check-Ins: Periodically reassess your goals, habits, and progress to ensure you're on track.

15. Adjust When Necessary: If you notice your progress slowing down, consider making strategic adjustments to your routine, whether it's in your diet or exercise.

16. Stay Positive: Maintain a positive outlook and focus on the benefits of a healthy lifestyle beyond just physical appearance.

CHAPTER FIVE

TAILORING THE DIET TO YOUR NEEDS

Adapting Metabolic Confusion for Dietary Restrictions

Adapting the metabolic confusion approach to dietary restrictions requires careful planning and creativity to ensure you meet your nutritional needs while still following the principles of the diet. Here's how you can modify the metabolic confusion diet to accommodate common dietary restrictions:

1. Vegetarian or Vegan:

- Protein Sources: Replace animal-based proteins with plant-based alternatives such as beans, lentils, chickpeas, tofu, tempeh, seitan, quinoa, nuts, and seeds.
- Omega-3s: Include sources of plant-based omega-3 fatty acids like flaxseeds, chia seeds, walnuts, and algae-based supplements.
- B12 and Iron: Monitor your intake of vitamin B12 and iron, as these nutrients are often lower in vegetarian or vegan diets. Consider fortified foods or supplements if necessary.

2. Gluten-Free:

- Grains: opt for gluten-free whole grains like rice, quinoa, millet, and certified gluten-free oats.
- Flours: Use gluten-free flours like almond flour, coconut flour, and chickpea flour for cooking and baking.
- Label Reading: Be diligent about reading labels to avoid hidden sources of gluten in packaged foods.

3. Dairy-Free:

- Calcium: Include fortified dairy-free milk alternatives (such as almond milk, soy milk, or oat milk) to ensure adequate calcium intake.
- Non-Dairy Yogurt: Choose non-dairy yogurt made from coconut, almond, soy, or cashew.
- Healthy Fats: Incorporate alternative sources of healthy fats like avocados, nuts, seeds, and olive oil.

4. Nut or Seed Allergies:

- Proteins: Rely on non-nut and non-seed sources of protein such as lean meats, poultry, fish, dairy (if not allergic), legumes, and gluten-free grains.
- Healthy Fats: Choose healthy fats from sources like avocados, olive oil, and coconut oil.

5. **Specific Allergies or Sensitivities:**

- Substitutions: Identify suitable substitutes for allergenic foods in recipes. For example, use sunflower seed butter if you are allergic to peanuts or almonds.
- Consult a Professional: Work with a dietitian to ensure you're getting all essential nutrients despite your dietary restrictions.

6. **Medical Conditions (e.g., Diabetes, High Blood Pressure):**

- Carbohydrates: Monitor carbohydrate intake and choose complex carbs to manage blood sugar levels.
- Sodium Intake: Choose low-sodium options and limit processed foods to manage blood pressure.

7. **Other Dietary Restrictions:**

- Research and Planning: Research recipes and resources that cater to your specific dietary needs and restrictions.
- Experiment with new foods and cooking methods to expand your options.

Strategies for Overcoming Challenges

Overcoming challenges while following the metabolic confusion diet, or any dietary plan, is an important part of achieving long-term success. Here are strategies to address common challenges and stay on track:

1. Cravings and Temptations:

- Plan for occasional treats and enjoy them mindfully.
- Keep healthier alternatives on hand when cravings strike.
- Use portion control to satisfy cravings without derailing progress.

2. Social Events and Eating Out:

- Check the menu in advance and make healthier choices.
- Eat a balanced meal or snack before attending an event to avoid overindulging.
- Opt for grilled, baked, or steamed options and ask for sauces or dressings on the side.

3. Time Constraints:

- Prepare meals and snacks in advance to have healthy options readily available.

- Opt for quick and easy recipes or use meal delivery services.

4. **Boredom or Lack of Motivation:**

    - Vary your meals and exercise routine to keep things interesting.
    - Set new goals and track your progress to stay motivated.

5. **Plateaus:**

    - Reassess your caloric intake and exercise routine to break through plateaus.
    - Change up your workout intensity, type, or duration.

6. **Emotional Eating:**

    - Practice mindfulness and identify triggers for emotional eating.
    - Find non-food ways to cope with emotions, such as going for a walk or practicing deep breathing.

7. **Lack of Support:**

    - Communicate your goals to friends and family, asking for their understanding and support.
    - Seek out online communities or support groups focused on your dietary plan.

8. **Traveling:**

- Pack healthy snacks and choose nutritious options while on the go.
- Research restaurants and grocery stores at your destination to make healthier choices.

9. **Stress:**

Engage in stress-reduction techniques like meditation, yoga, or deep breathing.

Prioritize self-care to manage stress levels.

10. **Lack of Time for Exercise:**

- Incorporate short bouts of exercise throughout the day, such as walking or bodyweight exercises.
- Choose efficient workouts like HIIT that provide maximum benefits in a short time.

11. **Plate Prep and Cooking Skills:**

- Invest time in learning simple cooking techniques and gradually build your skills.
- Explore meal prep strategies to save time during the week.

12. **Financial Constraints:**

- Focus on affordable, nutrient-dense foods like beans, lentils, whole grains, and seasonal produce.
- Buy in bulk when possible, to save money.

13. Fear of Failure:

- Embrace setbacks as learning opportunities rather than failures.
- Set realistic goals and celebrate small achievements along the way.

CHAPTER SIX

LIFESTYLE FACTORS FOR ENHANCED METABOLISM

Importance of Sleep for Metabolism

Sleep plays a crucial role in regulating various physiological processes, including metabolism. Getting adequate and quality sleep is essential for maintaining a healthy metabolism and overall well-being.

1. Energy Regulation:

- Sleep helps regulate the balance between energy intake (calories consumed) and energy expenditure (calories burned).
- Lack of sleep can disrupt this balance, leading to overeating and weight gain.

2. Hormonal Balance:

- Sleep influences the release of hormones that play a key role in metabolism, including insulin, cortisol, and leptin.
- Disrupted sleep patterns can lead to insulin resistance, increased cortisol (the stress hormone) levels, and disrupted appetite regulation.

3. **Appetite Regulation:**

- Sleep deprivation can lead to imbalances in the hormones ghrelin and leptin, which regulate hunger and fullness.
- Lack of sleep often leads to increased ghrelin (an appetite-stimulating hormone) and decreased leptin (a satiety hormone), causing overeating.

4. **Muscle Recovery and Growth:**

- Sleep is essential for muscle repair and growth, which are important for maintaining a higher metabolic rate.
- Growth hormone, which supports muscle development, is released during deep sleep.

5. **Restoring Cellular Function:**

- Sleep allows cells to repair and regenerate, maintaining proper metabolic function.
- During sleep, the body repairs and restores tissues, which contributes to overall metabolic health.

6. **Thermoregulation:**

- Sleep helps regulate body temperature, which is linked to metabolic rate.

- Poor sleep can disrupt temperature regulation and potentially impact metabolism.

7. **Circadian Rhythms:**

    - Adequate sleep is important for maintaining a healthy circadian rhythm, which influences the timing of metabolic processes.
    - Disruptions to circadian rhythms, such as irregular sleep patterns, can affect metabolism.

8. **Fat Metabolism:**

    - Sleep is involved in regulating the body's use of fats for energy.
    - Sleep deprivation may lead to impaired fat metabolism and storage, contributing to weight gain.

9. **Overall Health:** Chronic sleep deprivation is associated with a higher risk of obesity, type 2 diabetes, cardiovascular diseases, and other metabolic disorders.

10. **Stress Reduction:** Adequate sleep helps lower stress levels, which can contribute to a healthier metabolism and reduced inflammation.

11. Brain Health: Sleep is essential for cognitive function and decision-making, which can impact food choices and lifestyle behaviors.

12. Recovery from Exercise:

- Sleep is crucial for post-exercise recovery, allowing the body to repair muscle tissue and replenish energy stores.
- Prioritizing sleep is essential for maintaining a healthy metabolism and overall health. Aim for 7-9 hours of quality sleep per night, establish a regular sleep schedule, create a relaxing bedtime routine, and create a sleep-conducive environment to support your metabolic well-being.

Managing Stress and Its Impact on Aging

Managing stress is crucial for promoting healthy aging and overall well-being. Chronic stress can have a significant impact on various physiological processes and contribute to the aging process.

Impact of Stress on Aging:

1. Cellular Aging: Chronic stress can accelerate cellular aging by shortening telomeres, the protective caps at the ends of chromosomes. Shortened telomeres are associated with age-related diseases.

2. **Inflammation:** Stress triggers inflammation, which is linked to various age-related conditions, including cardiovascular diseases, diabetes, and cognitive decline.

3. **Hormonal Changes:** Prolonged stress can disrupt hormone balance, leading to increased cortisol levels. Elevated cortisol is associated with negative health outcomes and can contribute to metabolic issues.

4. **Cognitive Decline:** Chronic stress may contribute to cognitive decline and memory problems over time.

5. **Immune System:** Stress weakens the immune system's response, making individuals more susceptible to infections and illnesses.

Strategies for Managing Stress:

1. Practice mindfulness and meditation:

- Mindfulness and meditation techniques can help reduce stress and promote relaxation.
- These practices improve emotional regulation and increase resilience to stressors.

2. Physical Activity: Regular exercise helps release endorphins, natural mood lifters that combat stress.

- Engage in activities you enjoy, whether it's walking, yoga, swimming, or dancing.

3. Healthy Diet:

- Consume a balanced diet rich in fruits, vegetables, whole grains, lean proteins, and healthy fats.
- Nutrient-rich foods support the body's stress response and overall health.

4. Adequate Sleep:

- Prioritize quality sleep to support stress reduction and overall well-being.
- Aim for 7-9 hours of sleep each night.

5. Social Support:

- Maintain connections with friends and family members for emotional support.
- Share your feelings with loved ones to alleviate stress.

6. Time Management:

- Manage your time effectively to avoid feeling overwhelmed.
- Break tasks into manageable segments and prioritize them.

7. **Breathing Exercises:** Practice deep breathing exercises to trigger the relaxation response and reduce stress.

8. **Limit caffeine and alcohol:** Excessive caffeine and alcohol consumption can exacerbate stress and disrupt sleep patterns.

9. **Engage in Hobbies:** Pursue hobbies you enjoy to divert your focus from stressors and promote relaxation.

10. **Mind-Body Practices:** Engage in activities like tai chi, qigong, or progressive muscle relaxation that promote relaxation and mind-body connection.

11. **Professional Help:** If stress becomes overwhelming, consider seeking guidance from a therapist or counselor.

12. **Limit media exposure:** Set boundaries on media consumption, particularly news that can contribute to stress.

13. **Practice Gratitude:** Focus on the positive aspects of your life and practice gratitude daily.

Managing stress effectively is essential for promoting healthy aging and maintaining your overall health. By adopting stress management strategies and creating a balanced lifestyle, you can mitigate the negative effects of stress and enhance your well-being as you age.

CHAPTER SEVEN

TRACKING PROGRESS AND ADJUSTMENTS

Setting Realistic Goals for Health and Wellness

Setting realistic goals for health and wellness is crucial for creating sustainable changes and achieving long-term success. Unrealistic goals can lead to frustration and discouragement, while achievable goals can provide motivation and a sense of accomplishment. Here's how to set realistic goals:

1. Be Specific: Clearly define what you want to achieve. Avoid vague goals like "get healthy" and instead specify actions like "exercise three times a week."

2. Break down larger goals: If you have a big goal, break it into smaller, achievable steps. This makes the process more manageable and less overwhelming.

3. Make them measurable: Create goals that can be tracked and measured. This allows you to gauge your progress and make necessary adjustments.

4. Set Attainable Goals: Choose goals that are challenging but still within reach. Setting overly ambitious goals can lead to burnout.

5. Set short-term and long-term goals: Combine short-term goals (days to weeks) with long-term goals (months to years) for a balanced approach.

6. Use the SMART criteria: SMART stands for specific, measurably achievable, relevant, and time-bound. Applying these criteria helps ensure your goals are well-defined and achievable.

7. Focus on Behavior, Not Outcomes: Concentrate on actions and behaviors rather than outcomes you can't directly control. For instance, focus on eating more vegetables instead of losing a specific amount of weight.

8. Consider Your Lifestyle: Ensure your goals fit into your daily life and routines. A realistic goal should be something you can consistently incorporate.

9. Set Process and Outcome Goals: Combine process goals (actions you take) with outcome goals (results you want). This provides a well-rounded approach.

10. Celebrate Small Wins: Celebrate your achievements along the way, even if they're small steps toward your larger goal.

11. Reevaluate and Adjust: Regularly reassess your goals to ensure they're still relevant and adjust them as needed.

12. Stay Patient: Understand that progress takes time. Be patient and consistent in your efforts.

13. Focus on Health, Not Perfection: Aim for progress and better health rather than perfection or a specific appearance.

14. Be Flexible: Life is unpredictable. Be open to adapting your goals based on changing circumstances.

Setting realistic health and wellness goals helps you create a roadmap for achieving the changes you want to make. By breaking down your goals, tracking your progress, and making adjustments as needed, you increase your chances of successfully improving your well-being over the long term.

Identifying Plateaus and Making Necessary Changes

Plateaus are common in health and wellness journeys and occur when progress seems to stall despite your efforts. Identifying plateaus and making necessary changes is essential to continue moving toward your goals.

1. **Monitor Progress:** Regularly track your progress using measurements, photos, fitness benchmarks, and how you feel overall.

2. **Identify Patterns:** Look for trends in your progress. If you notice a consistent lack of change over several weeks, you might be experiencing a plateau.

3. **Evaluate Nutrition:** Reassess your dietary habits. Are you consistently following your chosen eating pattern? Are portion sizes accurate?

4. **Review Exercise Routine:** Analyze your workout routine. Have you been doing the same exercises at the same intensity for an extended period?

5. **Check Sleep and Stress:** Evaluate your sleep quality and stress levels. Inadequate sleep and chronic stress can hinder progress.

6. **Change Intensity:** Increase the intensity of your workouts. Add more weight, try interval training, or increase the duration of your sessions.

7. **Vary Exercises:** Introduce new exercises to challenge different muscle groups and prevent adaptation.

8. Modify Reps and Sets: Adjust the number of repetitions and sets for resistance exercises to challenge your muscles differently.

9. Adjust Cardiovascular Workouts: Alter the duration, intensity, and type of cardio workouts to avoid a plateau.

10. Nutrition Adjustments: If your progress has stalled, consider adjusting your calorie intake or macronutrient ratios based on your goals.

11. Try a Rest Week: Incorporate a week of lower-intensity workouts to allow your body to recover and reset.

12. Change the Routine: Alter your exercise routine entirely by trying a different type of fitness class or sport.

13. Review Nutritional Quality: Ensure your diet is balanced and nutrient-dense. Focus on whole foods and limit processed items.

14. Avoid Overtraining: Ensure you're allowing adequate time for recovery. Overtraining can lead to plateaus and even regression.

15. Stay Patient: Plateaus are a normal part of the process. Stay patient and remain committed to your goals.

16. Celebrate Non-Scale Victories: Look beyond the numbers on the scale and celebrate other achievements like improved strength or energy levels.

CHAPTER EIGHT

LONG-TERM MAINTENANCE AND BEYOND

Transitioning to a Sustainable Dietary Pattern

Transitioning to a sustainable dietary pattern is a long-term approach that focuses on creating a balanced and enjoyable way of eating that you can maintain over time. Here's how to make a smooth transition:

1. Reflect on Your Goals: Consider your health goals, preferences, and values. Your new dietary pattern should align with these aspects.

2. Gradual Changes: Avoid drastic shifts. Make small, gradual changes to your eating habits over time.

3. Prioritize Whole Foods: Emphasize whole, minimally processed foods like fruits, vegetables, lean proteins, whole grains, and healthy fats.

4. Balanced Meals: Create balanced meals that include a mix of carbohydrates, proteins, and fats to support your energy needs.

5. Mindful Eating: Practice mindful eating by paying attention to hunger and fullness cues. Eat slowly and savor your meals.

6. Hydration: Drink plenty of water throughout the day to support digestion and overall health.

7. Portion Control: Focus on portion control to avoid overeating. Listen to your body's signals of fullness.

8. Include Treats Mindfully: Allow yourself occasional treats or foods you enjoy, but consume them mindfully and in moderation.

9. Meal Planning: Plan your meals and snacks in advance to make healthier choices more convenient.

10. Diversity and Variety: Include a variety of foods to ensure you're getting a wide range of nutrients. Experiment with different recipes and cuisines.

11. Listen to Your Body: Pay attention to how different foods make you feel. Adjust your diet based on how your body responds.

12. Learn Cooking Skills: Enhance your cooking skills to create delicious and nutritious meals at home.

13. Minimize Added Sugars and Processed Foods: Gradually reduce your intake of sugary foods and highly processed items.

14. Focus on Fiber: Incorporate fiber-rich foods like whole grains, fruits, vegetables, and legumes to support digestion and satiety.

15. Regular Check-Ins: Periodically assess how you feel, your energy levels, and any changes in your body.

16. Celebrate Progress: Celebrate your successes, whether they're small improvements in your eating habits or larger health achievements.

CONCLUSION

In conclusion, the journey towards improved health, well-being, and sustainable vitality is a dynamic and multifaceted endeavor. Throughout our exploration of the "Metabolic Confusion Diet for Seniors" and related topics, we've delved into the intricate interplay of metabolism, aging, nutrition, exercise, stress management, and lifestyle choices. By synthesizing this knowledge, we can create a holistic perspective that empowers us to make informed decisions for our long-term health.

We've learned that metabolism, the complex engine that powers our bodies, undergoes changes as we age. These changes are influenced by various factors, including genetics, lifestyle, and hormonal shifts. The "Metabolic Confusion Diet for Seniors" offers a strategic approach that leverages variation in exercise and nutrition to stimulate metabolism and promote healthy aging. By embracing this approach, seniors can harness the power of metabolic confusion to optimize their well-being and maintain a vibrant lifestyle.

Crucially, a balanced diet rich in nutrient-dense foods, portion control, and mindful eating forms the cornerstone of this dietary strategy. By providing our bodies with the right fuel, we can sustain energy levels, support metabolic function, and foster healthy aging. Moreover, incorporating regular exercise routines that encompass cardiovascular, strength training, and flexibility exercises is key to maintaining muscle mass, bone density, and overall vitality.

However, this journey isn't just about diet and exercise—it extends to managing stress, prioritizing sleep, and cultivating a positive mindset. We've explored the profound impact of stress on aging and how practicing stress-reduction techniques contributes to our overall well-being. Adequate sleep, a vital component of a healthy lifestyle, plays an integral role in regulating metabolism, cognitive function, and emotional balance.

Transitioning to a sustainable dietary pattern involves setting realistic goals, embracing diversity in food choices, and integrating metabolic confusion principles into our daily lives. By gradually implementing these principles, we can create a lifestyle that supports our individual needs, preferences, and goals.

Ultimately, our journey towards health and well-being is a lifelong endeavor—one that requires patience, self-compassion, and a commitment to continuous learning and growth. The knowledge and strategies we've explored offer a roadmap to navigate the complexities of aging and metabolism, empowering us to make informed choices that promote vitality, longevity, and an enriched quality of life.

As we move forward, let us carry with us the understanding that our bodies are remarkable vessels, capable of adaptation and transformation. By embracing the principles of the "Metabolic Confusion Diet for Seniors" and integrating them into our unique journeys, we embark on a path of empowerment, resilience, and well-being that honors the gift of a healthy and fulfilling life.

Made in the USA
Columbia, SC
30 August 2023

1bdbdb0c-8070-424c-a71d-15e15e866c20R02